THE ART OF THE DISPENSATION

(Basic orientations for the correct use of the medicines)

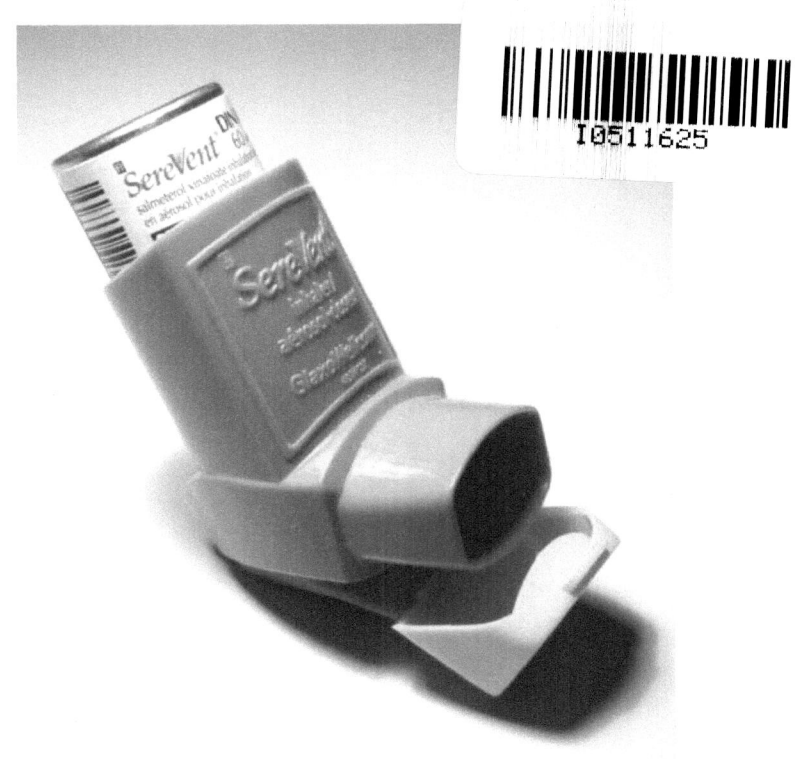

JUAN E. CALDERIN CAMPBELL

If you want different results
don't continuous doing the same...

ALBERT EINSTEN

PREFACE

The extraordinary relevance of the pharmaceutical industry in the current world and the impact of new drugs in the world population stuck to the human necessity of maintaining the health especially for the subsistence in the capitalist societies, they have incentivized in people the medication as a normal habit in their lifestyle either with medical goals, or for pleasure, sport practice or for aesthetic practice.

It is necessary to say that this medication in a great number of cases lacks medical orientation reason why we should talk about self-medication terms, which is in my approach; the most extended related drugs problem all over the world.

The present book has as objective to impel the divulgation about the dispensation practice on the management of the medications and to contribute a didactic instrument to satisfy the necessities of knowledge on the manipulation and administration of the drugs.

This book allows us from a comprehensive panoramic to contemplate through the pharmaceutical forms or the pharmacological groups which are the requirements or necessary instructions for their correct use.

The knowledge is distributed describing in a simple but comprehensible modest way the topics they are the most remarkable in the daily life of a patient.

I want to specify that all the abreviations that appears in this book has been taken from the official school of pharmacy of Pontevedra which has been described in the references number 14,15 and 16 in this book. In this description the reader can find also the electronic address of this information.

As author, I would like to express my gratitude and my satisfaction for to put in the hands of students and my colleagues these pages which I consider very important in order to give education to our patients and with this education, to contribute to increase their quality of life.

Juan E. Calderín Campbell

Table of content

correct use of the homeopathy/ 1
correct use of the aromatherapy/ 3
correct use of the flower therapy/ 5
correct use of the aerosols/ 7
correct use of the suppositories/ 9
The correct use of the antibiotics./ 12
correct use of the ear drops/ 14
correct use of the eyes drops/ 15
The correct use of the nasal drops/ 17
The correct use of the psychoactives drugs/ 19
The correct use of the suspentions/ 21
Pessaries and vaginal tablets/ 23
The correct use of te antiparasitary medicines/ 25
The correct use of the antialergic and the antiasmatic medicines/ 27
The correct use of the insulin / 28
The injection of the intramuscular penicillin/ 30
Correct use of the oftalmic ointment / 34
The correct use of the local anestethic in gel presentation (for to apply in the anus) / 36
The correct use of the suspentions for reconstitution solvents solutions / 38
the correct use of the analgesics in a semisolid formulation/ 39

The correct use of the powdered nutritional supplement/ 41

The correct use of the oral rehiadratation salts (ORS)/ 42

The correct use of the sun protection cream/ 44

The correct use of the birth-control pills or family planning pills/ 45

I)- CORRECT USE OF THE HOMEOPATHY.

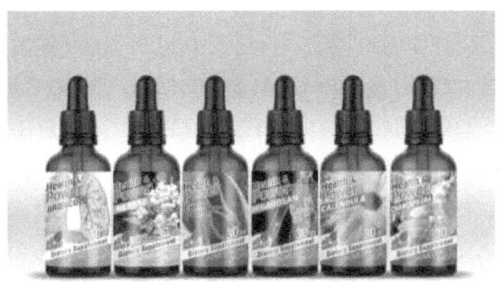

Picture # 1. It represents some homeopathy medications.

The homeopathy is a therapeutic method directed to the prevention, relief or cure of illnesses and that is used for this work the medicines that we use as homeopathic medicines.

This type of treatment has demonstrated effectiveness for the prevention and treatment of diverse illnesses like the flu, cough, diarrhea, migraine crisis, bruises, that is to say the one that we know as acute illnesses and chronic illnesses as the allergy, the dermatitis, the asthma, rheumatic affections, anxiety and other pathologies.

Presentation forms: Drops.

The homeopathic medicines has the great advantage that, they don't present contraindications or interactions with other medicines neither greats adverse effects with the industrial medicines that the patients use to buy in the pharmacies.

USE AND CORRECT PROCEDURE FOR THE HOMEOPATHIC MEDICINES

1. Is recommended to the patient that must be informed and updated firstly on this type of medication with a specialized doctor.
2. If you as patient have some base treatment should communicate immediately to their head doctor that will start with another type of treatment to guarantee in this way the consensus between professionals and their advises.
3. The patient must keep in mind that must not exchange the industrial medicine that is scientifically proven and of obligatory use in many cases as the antibiotics or to treat serious illnesses of urgency illnesses.
4. As in every medication the dose should be respected and progressive only under medical criteria.

5. This should be taken 15 minutes before the foods or with the empty stomach.

6. To keep in mind the general rules for the use of the medicines.

II)- CORRECT USE OF THE AROMATHERAPY

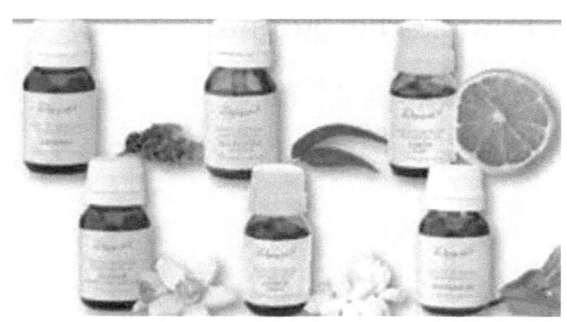

Picture # 2. It represents a kit of some of the essential oils more used in the treatment with aromatherapy.

The aromatherapy is a branch of the herbal medicine that exercises its functions by the use of the vegetable oils. This is summarized in that there is a previous process of extraction of the essential oils contents in vegetable drugs are used in diverse forms as the bath, compresses, inhalations, masks, creams and massages with therapeutic goals that reside in to improve the physical, mental health or both of them. Maybe their biggest particularity is that these are not ingested but rather they are inhaled or are applied on the skin.

Presentation forms: Drops.

USE AND CORRECT PROCEDURE FOR THE OILS ESSENTIAL IN AROMATHERAPY

1. The dose indicated by the doctor should not be violated.
2. The patient should know the therapeutic effects of each essential oil because as the immense majority of the existent medications, the essential oils each one of them have a different therapeutic action.
3. The essential oils should be diluted in some substance in order to diminish its effect. These substances can be water, vegetable oils, clays and hidrolatos, among others.
4. The essential oils are very concentrated and they should not be applied directly in the skin.
5. To keep in mind the general rules for the correct use of the medications.

III)- CORRECT USE OF THE FLOWER THERAPY

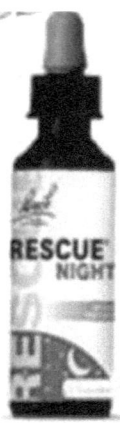

Picture # 3. It represents a rescue flask that means rescue. A medication of the floral therapy frequently used against the stress and the insomnia by this cause.

It is well known in the whole world the existence and application of this therapy.

Their therapeutic objective is based on achieving the emotional balance by the use of the essences.

Is necessary to understand that these are not more than solutions of natural substances and not properly drgus.

Presentation forms: Drops

THE CORRECT USE OF THE FLOWER THERAPY

1. The application of this therapy should be carried out the under the doctor's low supervision.
2. It is recommended to add 2 drops from the chosen flower to a glass of mineral water that the patient must take during the day, as often as it is necessary, a minimum of 4 times, separated from the foods.
3. As a characteristic that distinguishes it of any other treatment this treatment does not have a limit of time for to end because the application of this therapy depends of the emotional status of the patient.
4. To keep in mind the general rules for the correct use of the medicines.

IV)- USE CORRECT OF THE AEROSOLS

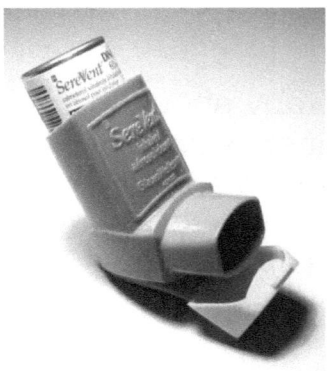

Picture # 4. This picture represents a device, an inhaler of the aerosol coupled to the flask of the medicine in pressurized form.

Presentation forms: Generally metallic pressurized recipient.

THE USE CORRECT OF THE AEROSOLS

1. After expectorating the most as possible, the capsule should be placed according to the instructions in the leaflet, the air should be expelled emptying the lungs slowly as much as it is possible and the inhaler should be introduced in the mouth, then keeping the

lips strongly together around it, the head should be leans lightly back and then the patient should inspired Deeply through the inhaler, after this step the patient must controls the breathing from 10 to 15 seconds and later must exhaled the air through the nose and lastly the mouth is rinsed with lukewarm water.

2. If this procedure is not adequate technique diminishes the effect of the drug and it drives to therapeutic failure.

V)- THE CORRECT USE OF THE SUPPOSITORIES

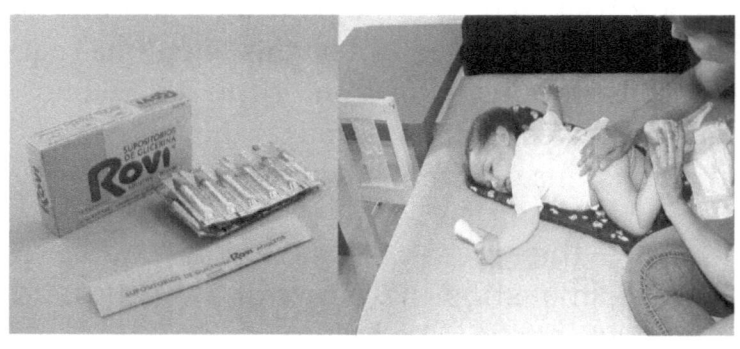

A   B

Picture # 5. It shows two you imagines. A and B.

A) – This picture shows the container of the medicine and the blister that contains the suppositories.

B) - A mother carrying out the placement procedure of the suppository to the baby.

(We can see that she maintains the gluteus closes to avoid the expulsion of the medicine).

Presentation forms: Blister of aluminum paper or plastic.

THE USE CORRECT OF THE SUPPOSITORIES

1. To wash well the hands be with water and soap before and after the application of the suppository.

Note: This procedure avoids that the mother or tutor or who is the applicator of the medicines can transmit an anal parasitic, a bacteria or herpes to the baby.

2 - The suppositories should not be fractioned because the quantity of active principles will never be the same because the head of the suppository is bigger than the rest of the suppository, in the case that the dose require to cut it, the patient or care giver should cut it in a longitudinal way.

3 - If it happens, the expulsion of the suppository, before the first three minutes after the insertion, then the patient can put a new one, but if the expiltion occurs more than 10 minutes after the insertion, the patient must not insert a new one because a part of the dose was already absorbed and the new one can means an overdose.

Note: the exception of this rule are the suppository of glicerine because these suppositories does not have active principles, they are just a lubricant substance.

VI) - THE CORRECT USE OF THE ANTIBIOTICS.

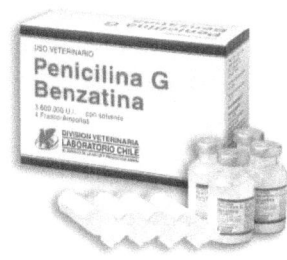

Figure # 6. This picture shows the container with the vials of penicillin and the water for injection.

Presentation forms: In all the pharmaceutical forms.

THE USE CORRECT OF THE ANTIBIOTICS

1 – Don't drink alcohol or any drink that contains alcohol.

2 - If you don't improve in the next 7 days after to start the treatment you must go to see the doctor immediately.

3 –If you feel better at the half of time of the treatment don't stop and finish the treatment in the correct way as the doctor says for to avoid the reinfection or resurgence of the bacteria.

Note: these rules are general for all the antibiotics. Every medicine are adapted to the specifies of them and the leaflet.

VII- CORRECT USE OF THE EAR DROPS

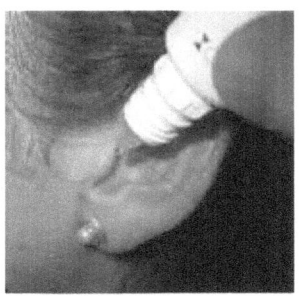

Picture # 7. This picture shows the procedure of instillation of the ear drops in the patient's ear.

Presentation forms: Plastic recipients of 5 to 10 ml.

THE USE CORRECT OF THE EAR DROPS

1-To wash well the hands.
2-To hold the flask in the hand for several minutes until to reach an appropriate temperature, around 40,6 centigrade degrees
3-To lean the head or to go to bed of side.
4-straighten the auditory conduct taking the superior part of the auricular pavilion and to throw of it smoothly up and behind in the adults, in the case of the children the lobe should be thrown down and behind.
5-To apply the quantity of medicine prescribed by the doctor and to wait approximately 5 minutes before being turned for the application of the medicine in the other ear.

VIII)-CORRECT USE OF THE EYES DROPS

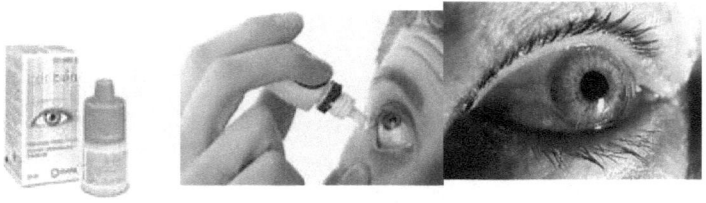

A   B   C

Picture # 8. This picture shows.
A)-Container with the recipient of the eye drop.
B)-Procedure of instillation of the eye drops in the conjuntival sack.
C) – A human eye that suffers a conjunctivitis type.

Presentation forms: Plastic recipients of 5 to 10 ml.

THE CORRECT USE OF THE EYE DROPS

1 – To wash well the hands.

2 –Don't touch the tip or cover of the dropper.
3- To look up.
4 -To throws down the inferior lid to make a sack.

5 – You must put the tip of the dropper as close as possible from the eye but the tip must not touch the eye.

6 - To instill the drop.

7 - To close the lids smoothly during 1 or 2 minutes (not very strong) and to dry the excess of the medicine in the external part of the eye.

IX) - THE CORRECT USE OF THE NASAL DROPS

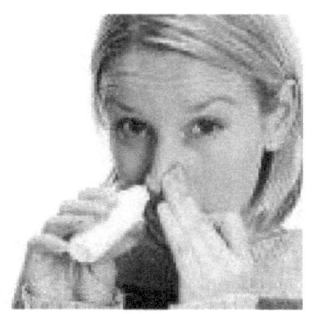

Figure # 9. The image shows a patient in one of the steps for the installation of a nasal drop. (Steps 3 and 4).

Presentation forms: flasks of 5 to 10 ml.

THE USE CORRECT OF THE NASAL DROPS.

1 - The head the most extended back as possible or to lie in the bed face up or with a pillow under the shoulders.
2 - To shake the spray - it can be a plastic flask for leak - to insert the tip in a nasal grave of our chosen.
3 - To cover the other nasal grave one and to close the mouth.
4 - To apply the spray and to aspire slowly in a

simultaneous way and to retire the applicator and to bend toward before until to put the head between the knees and then to breath throw the mouth for some seconds.

X) - THE CORRECT USE OF THE PSYCHOACTIVES DRUGS

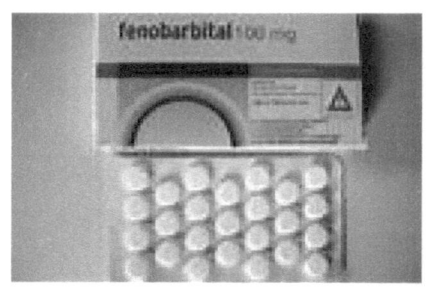
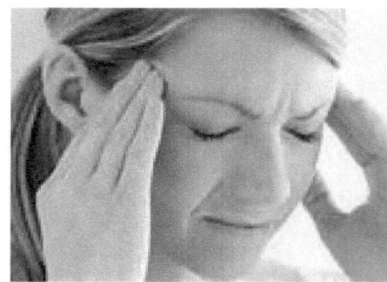

A   B

Picture # 10. This picture shows:

A) The container and recipient in this case a blister of phenobarbital 100 mg a famous psychoactive drug.
B) Patient that suffers psychosis, pathology of the nervous system.

Presentation forms: blíster x 20 pills of 100 mg each one.

THE CORRECT USE OF THE PSYCHOACTIVES DRUGS

1 - Do not drink alcoholic drinks during the treatment.

2 - Do not to drive vehicles neither to operate machineries where a decrease of the attention can originate accidents.

3 – To read often the leaflet.

4 – Try to be advised by another person in case the mental status can be worse because among other things you can make a mistake in the doses during you are under treatment.

XI- THE CORRECT USE OF THE SUSPENTIONS

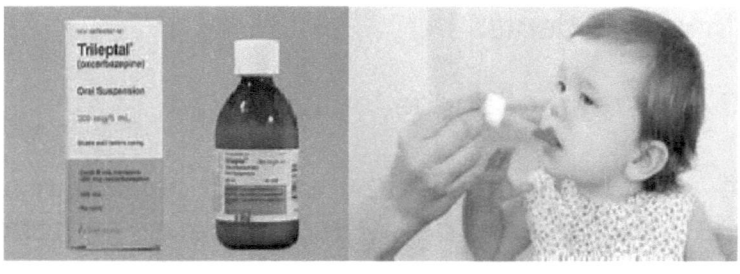

A   B

Picture # 11. This picture shows:

A) The container and recipient in this case a flask of 120 ml that contains the medication as powder for reconstitution as a suspention.

B) Administration of the dose to a pediatric patient using a dropper.

Presentation forms: flask of 120 ml.

THE CORRECT USE OF THE SUSPENTIONS

1 - To boil well the water.

2 - To add the water to the flask with the powder for suspension until the half.

3 - To shake until complete disillusion.

4 - To complete the volume of the flask until the shoulders avoiding the contact among the liner (internal cover of the cover and the solution).

5 – To shake the container for 1 minute before to administrate the medicine to the patient according to the dosage indicated by the physician.

6 - To conserve in refrigeration. (Just in controlled Temperature the medicine should not be freeze.

7-After seven days of the preparation you can consider the suspention expired.

XII-PESSARIES AND VAGINAL TABLETS

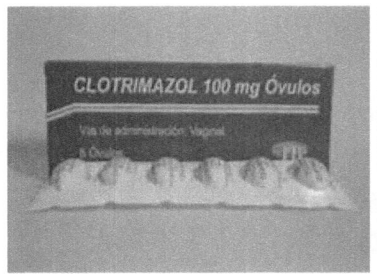 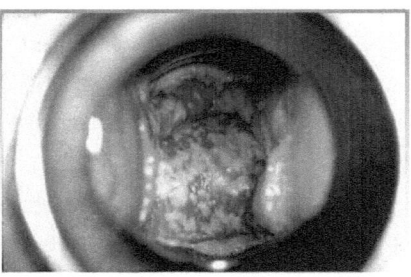

　　　　A　　　　　　　　B

Picture # 12. This picture shows:

A) The container and recipient in this case a blister with six pessaries of clotrimazol 100 mg.
B) The interior of a vagine with the secretions in an infectious process.

Presentation forms: Blister with six pessaries of clotrimazol 100 mg.

THE CORRECT USE OF THE PESSARIES AND THE VAGINAL TABLETS.

1 - To be wash the hands well.

2- To lie down in the bed face up and to open the legs.

2 - To place the pessary or the vaginal pill the as deepest as possible in the interior of the vagine.

2.1- The pessary can be collocate with the fingers.

2.2- If the patient is having an applicator must put the pessary in the applicator and to slide the applicator very carefully as deep as possible and to relieve the pessary slowly and later to retire the applicator).

3 - To stay lie down in the bed face up. (In the medical science we know this position as supine decubitus).

4 - To cover the external lips of the vagine with a sanitary clothe in order to avoid that the medicine go out.

5 –To wash well the hands at the end of the procedure.

6 - To keep the medicine in refrigeration according to the instructions of the leaflet or the container.

XIII-THE CORRECT USE OF TE ANTIPARASITARY MEDICINES.

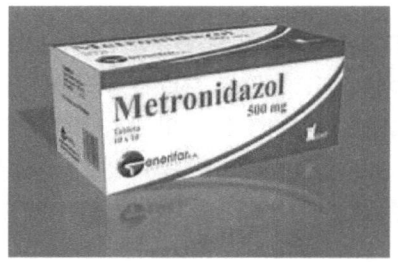 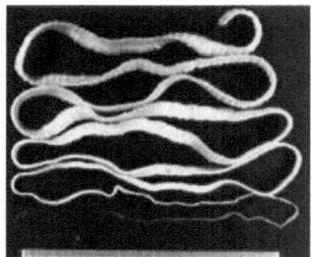

A   B

Figure # 13. This picture shows:

A) The container and recipient in this case a box of metronidazole (Fragil) 500 mg.

B) This picture represents the *Taenia solium* a parasitic that can live in the human bowels and van reach the 3 or 4 meters of length. This parasite can mortal for the children.

Presentation forms: Blister with 20 pills of 500 mg c/u.

THE CORRECT USE OF THE ANTIPARASITARICS

1 - To wash hands well.

2 - Do not drink alcoholic drinks.

3 – To take the medicine with the stomach empty, fasting or after the meals according to the leaflet or the medical orientation.

4 – To keep the medicine in the refrigerator in a controlled temperature according to the leaflet or the container's indication.

5 - To maintain the hygienic and sanitary measures. (To wash the vegetables well, to cook the foods well, and to wash well the hands after any procedure, etc.)

XIV- THE CORRECT USE OF THE ANTIALERGIC AND THE ANTIASMATIC MEDICINES

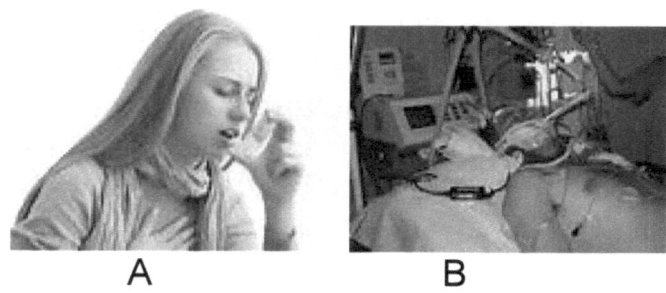

A   B

Picture # 14. This picture shows:

A) - A patient that is taking a dose of the inhaler.
B) - The picture shows a patient coupled to the artificial ventilation; after an asthmatic status.

THE CORRECT USE OF THE ANTIALERGICS AND ANTIASMATHICS DRUGS

1- To wash well the hands.
2 - Do not to ingest alcoholic drinks.
3- To take the medicines according to medical indication.
4 - To conserve the medicine in refrigeration or according to the indication of the leaflet or the container.

XIV- THE CORRECT USE OF THE INSULIN.

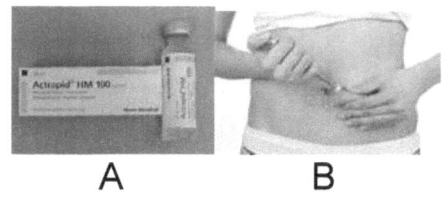

A   B

Picture # 15. This picture shows:

A. Avial of insulin ACTRAPID HM 100 units.
B. It shows of a patient administrating the insulin in the abdominal area itself.

THE CORRECT USE OF THE INSULIN

1 – To wash well the hands.

2 - To select the place of the injection well, to wash it well and to leave it dries off.

3 - To disinfect the skin with the antiseptic solution of alcohol 70%.

4 - To expel the air of the needle, to make a pleat in

the skin and to insert the needle in their base in an angle from 20 to 30 degrees, later, to liberate the pleat and to aspire shortly, if blood doesn't appear then the solution should be injected slowly and later the needle should be extracted quickly. Then massage is given with an antiseptic cloth or cotton. (If blood appears the patient should extract the needle immediately and to get another site of injection).

5 - To watch over their health status and to make sure of being in good condition for to injected the insulin.

6 - To fulfill the requirements for to administrate the medicine. (Do not to be traveling long distances, do not make physical exercises, do not to be pregnant or if the patient feels that can experience a hypoglycemic episode, etc.).

7 – To administrate the injection avoiding the contamination off the plastic syringe or the glass (In the case of the glass one it should be boiled for 15 minutes before to administrate the medicine.

8 – To administrate the insulin always taking into account the map of the body that we use for to inject the insulin.

XV- THE INJECTION OF THE INTRAMUSCULAR PENICILIN

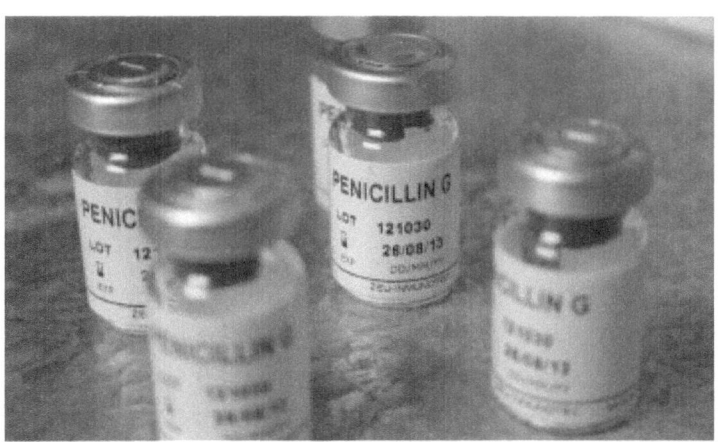

Picture # 16. The picture shows some vials of penicillin G for injection.

   1. The material for the procedure as the vials as and the water should be taken very carefully.
   2. The materials should be handle and should be prepared in a clean place.
   3. The correct status of the medicines should be cheked.
   4. To check the expire date for to be sure that the medicines are not expired.
   5. To wash well the hands.
   6. The person who handle the medicine should be

use latex gloves for their protection and for to avoid the contamination of the hands, the material and the medicines.

7. The person that manipulates the medicine as the one who will receive the medicine must not be allergic to the penicillin or to any other of its components of a similar chemical structure

8. To use a syringe that is not expired in its expiration date.

9. To check that the recipient of the syringe, plastic or nylon has been correctly sealed. (Some syringes bring from the factory a disinfectant alcoholic solution (we should be sure that this liquid has not been evaporated because it indicates the presence of microscopic pores)).

10. To extract the syringe with the care and purpose of maintaining the needle inside their protective container.

11. To revise that the needle is not this blunted.

12. To carry out the disinfection of the selected gluteus -the gluteus is selected in dependence of if it has been injected the previous time, among other approaches - with cotton with alcoholic disinfectant solution with circular movements from inside toward out.

13. To be sure that the syringe doesn't have air in its interior.

14. To extract the water for injection of the vial.

15. To uncover the aluminum cover that covers the vial of penicillin.
16. To insert the needle in the vial through the rubber cover.
17. To inject the water for injection in the vial.
18. To mix the water for injection with the contained powder in the vial shaking it.
19. To mix with movements of agitation and rotational in the hands until achieving the complete homogeneity of the mixture.
20. To puncture the vial through the rubber cover to carry out the extraction of the penicillin.
21. To extract the mixture from the vial with the care of not leaving medicine in the original recipient and with the caution that the syringe doesn't contain air in its interior.
22. To carry out a soft leak of the medicine through the needle in order to be sure that the needle is not obstructed by the medicine (this preparation is a suspension and it can precipitate quickly).
23. To divide the gluteus in four quadrants choosing with caution in the case of the right one, the right superior quadrant this is distant from the veins and the arteries.
24. To keep with the fingers the area of the gluteus that will be injected. (To make a pleat).
25. To insert the needle in the skin in an angle of 90 degrees.

26. To carry out an aspiration with the syringe to be sure that the needle does not break any vein or arteries.

27. If the medicine in the syringe adquire a red color is because the needle has broken a vein or arteries and then we should retire the needle and to start all the process again with another syringe and with another dose of the medicine

28. To inject the liquid of the medicine very slowly.

29. To take out the needle once finished the procedure in the same angle that it was introduced in the gluteus, to throw it away and to cover the injection point with dry cotton pressing smoothly.

30. To discard the material used in sure places, not the garbage.

XVII- CORRECT USE OF THE OFTALMIC OINTMENT

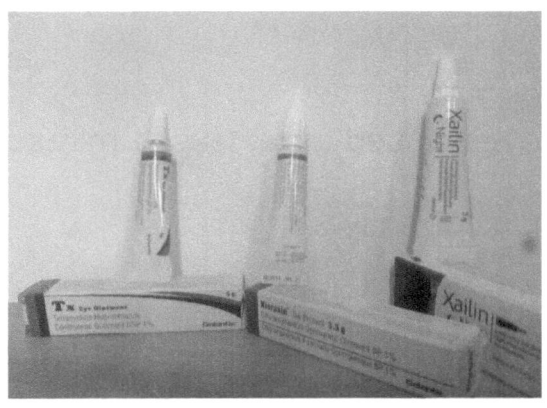

Picture # 17. This picture shows some ophthalmic ointments.

THE CORRECT USE OF THE OPHTHALMIC OINTMENTS

1 – To wash the hands correctly.
2 - To move away the cover that covers the aluminum tube.
3 - To apply a thin ribbon of the medicine deep in the conjuntival sack always avoiding to touch the pupil of the eye with the tip of the cover (When the tube of the medicine is at room temperature is more easy to apply the medicine).

4 – If the patient must to apply in the eye more than one medicine must wait at least 5 to 15 minutes between them in order to facilitate the correct absorption of the medicines.

5 – To cover the tube.
6 - To maintain the eyes closed for at least 1 minute after each application.
7 - To wash the hands correctly.

XVIII- THE CORRECT USE OF THE LOCAL ANESTETHIC IN GEL PRESENTATION (For to apply in the anus).

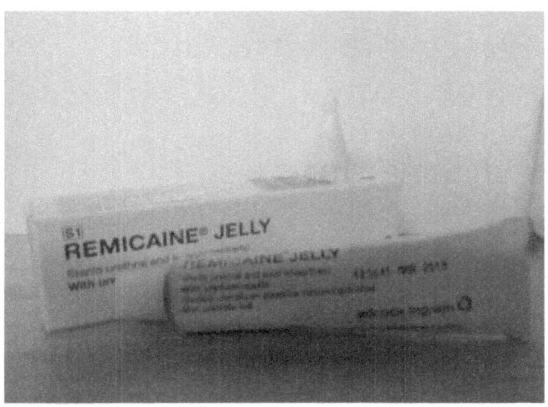

Picture # 18. This picture shows an analgesic gel.

THE CORRECT USE OF THE LOCAL ANALGESIC IN GEL PRESENTATION (For to apply in the anus).

1 - To wash the hands correctly.
2 - To apply the medicine in the fingers.
3 - To apply the gel smoothly on the anus.
4 - To wash the hands correctly.

　　　If the procedure takes part after the defecation the patient must fellow these steps.

5 - After the defecation to move away the remains with supreme care preferably washing without soap in order to avoid the presence of chemical substances contained in the formula of the soap that can be an irritating substance.
6 - To dry off with humid towel or with cotton.
7 - To wash well the hands.
8 - To apply the gel on the fingers.
9 - To apply smoothly on the anus.
10 - To wash the hands well.

XIX- THE CORRECT USE OF THE SUSPENTIONS FOR RECONSTITUTION SOLVENTS SOLUTIONS.

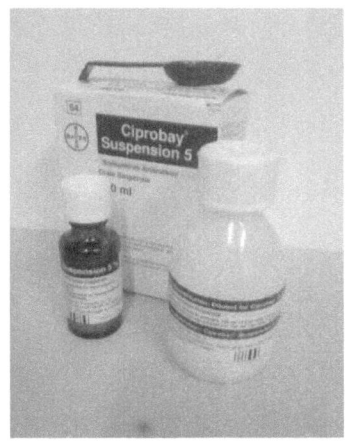

Picture # 19. The picture represents an antibiotic in suspension for reconstitution.

THE CORRECT USE OF THE SUSPENCIONES FOR RECONSTITUTION

1 – To wash the hands well.
2 - To add the liquid content to the solid.
3 - To shake the flask until complete the dissolution.
4 - To administrate the medicine to the patient according to the doctor's indication.

XX- THE CORRECT USE OF THE ANALGESICS IN A SEMISOLID FORMULATION

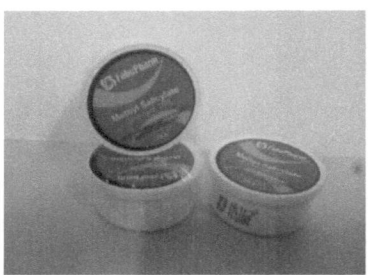

Picture # 20. This picture represents some containers Methylsalicilate.

THE CORRECT USE OF THE METYLSALICILATE

1 – To wash well the hands.
2 - To wash the area where the medicine will be apply.
3 - To apply well rubbing on the affected area.
4 – Must not be applyed on an open wound, or burned area or over the sensitive skin.
5 – To apply with special care in hipomelanics patients (albino).
6 - Not to rub in a rude way to avoid the burn during the friction.

7 – Must have extreme care during the application in the head because it can be crawled to the eyes throw the sweat.
8 - To wash the hands well after the application.

XXI- THE CORRECT USE OF THE POWDERED NUTRITIONAL SUPPLEMENT

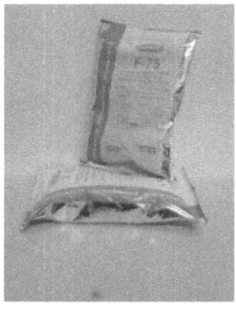

Figure # 21. This picture represents sachet of a nutritional supplement.

THE CORRECT USE OF THE POWDERED NUTRITIONAL SUPPLEMENT

1 - To wash the hands well.
2 - To boil a liter of water.
3 - To allow the water boiled until refreshing that is to say until arriving to the normal temperature.
4 - To take half liter of water.
5 - To pour on the content in the sachet in half liter of lukewarm water.
6 - To shake this mixture until complete dissolution.
7 - To administrate to the patient according to the dose indicated by the doctor.

XXII- THE CORRECT USE OF THE ORAL REHIADRATATION SALTS (ORS)

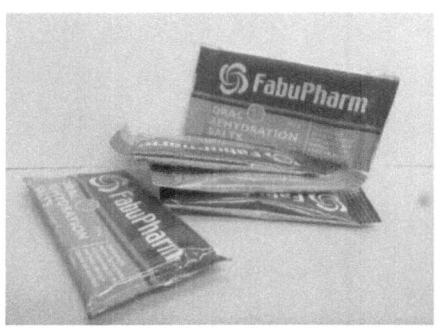

Figure # 22. The figure shows some sachets of Oral Rehidratation Salts.

THE CORRECT USE OF THE ORAL REHIDRATATION SALTS.

1 – To wash well the hands.
2 - To boil a liter of water.
3 - To allow the boiled water to rest and refresh until to reach the room temperature.
4 - To take half liter of water.
5 - To pour on the content of the sachet in half liter of lukewarm water and to shake the mixture until the complete dissolution.

7 - To administrate to the patient according to the dose indicated by the doctor.

XXIII- THE CORRECT USE OF THE SUN PROTECTION CREAM

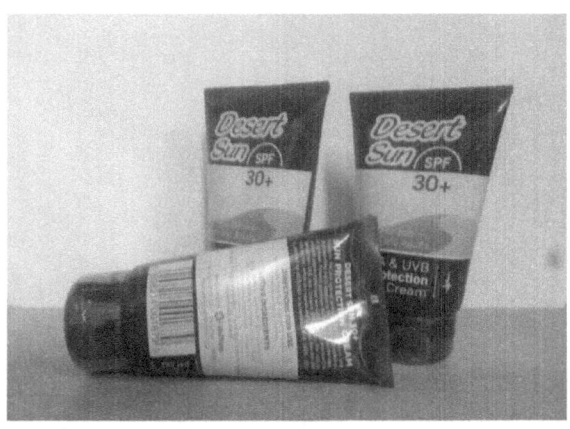

Figure # 23. This picture represents some tubes of the cream for the protection of the skin from the sun.

THE CORRECT USE OF THE CREAM FOR SOLAR PROTECTION

1- To wash well the hands.
2- To apply especially in the parts of the body that are most exposed to the sun.
3- It is recommended to the patient to use sun glasses and long sleeves clothes for the protection of the skin.

XXVII- THE CORRECT USE OF THE BIRTH-CONTROL PILLS OR FAMILY PLANNING PILLS

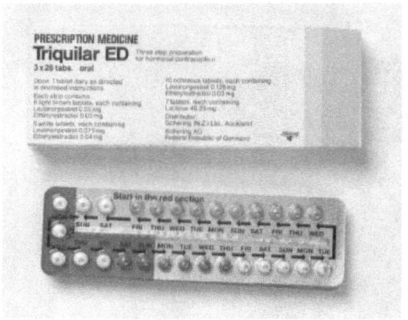

Figure # 27. This picture represents the birth-control pills of triquilar also known as Family Planning Pills.

The birth-control medications in general are manufactured with the final objective of achieving the non-conception of the pregnancy.

THE CORRECT USE OF THE BIRTH-CONTROL PILLS OR FAMILY PLANNING PILLS

1. The first pill should be taken the first day of the menstrual cycle and the patient must continuous taking the medicine without to interrupt the starting treatment from this date during the whole time that the birth-control effect is wanted.

2. The medicine should be taken at the same hour every day and always after the night food or before going to bed.

3. The interval between tablets must be 24 hours.

4. Must keep in mind that if this interval is superior to 27 hours the patient can lost the protection of the medicine.

5. The patient should know that the real birth-control effect begins after to take the tablet number 15 that's why during the first 14 days the patient must have protected sexual relations.

6. If exists a failure in the adherence, that is to say, if the patient forgets to take the medicine one day, then the patient should continue with both types of contraception until to take 14 pills again.

7. This medicine should not be taking until three or four weeks after the woman give birth, because

the effects of the medicine in the baby that the mother is breastfeeding are still ignored.

8. The woman that has taken this medicine previously and had allergy episodes must not take this medicine. For her this medicine is contraindicated and she should go to the doctor for a different prescription,

9. The nauseas, vomits and sickness are adverse reactions of this medicine. The patient should not confuse these symptoms with the symptoms of the pregnancy which are the same ones. If the patient is not sure of their good adherence to the medication then she must go to the doctor for specialized verification or carry out a pregnancy test.

ABREVIATIONS USED IN THE MEDICAL PRESCRIPTION

Abreviaturas usadas en las recetas médicas	
%	Per cent
a.c.	Before the meals
Aa	At equal parts
Ad tertian vicem	For three times
Ad. Lib.	As much as you wish (del latín: *ad libitum*)
Alt. dieb.	Alternative days (del latín: *alternis diebus*)
Alt. horis	Alternative hours (del latín: *alternis horis*)
Alt. noct.	Alternative nights (del latín *alternis noctibus*)
Amp	Ampules
b.i.d.	Twice a day (del latín: *bis in die*)
c.	with
c.c.	With meals (del latín: *cum cibis*)
c.m.	Tomorrow in the morning (del latín: *cras mane*)
c.n.	Tomorrow in the nigth (del latín: *cras nocte*)
c.s.	Enough quantity
Cap	Capsules
Co.	Compound (del latín: *compsitum*)
Coch.	Spoon
Coch. Med.	Median spoon of aproximately 8 ml
Cochleat.	By sponnfuls
Comp	Comprimide
d.s.a.	Disolve according to art.
Dieb. Tert.	Each three days, one day yes and two no (del latín: *diebus terttis*)
Dil.	Diluted (del latín: *dilue*)

e.m.p.	As prescription
Exc.	Excipient
f. o ft.	Make (del latín: *fiat*)
F.M.	Magistral formula
Gtt	Drop (s)
h.n.	This night (del latín: *hac nocte*)
h.s., hor. Som., QHS	At time to sleep
h.s.a.	Make according to art
In aq.	In water (del latín: *in aqua*)
In d.	Daily (del latín: *in dies*)
m.	Mix
m.d.u.	As it was indicated (del latín: *ut a me dictum*)
M.O.	Modus operandum
m.s.a.	Mix according to art
Man.	In the morning (del latín: *mane*)
Mit.	send (del latín: *mitte*)
N. o noct.	At night (del latín: *nocte*)
n. y m.	Night and morning (del latín: *nocte et mane*)
N.B.	Check well (del latín: *nota bene*)
o.d.	Right eye
O.l. y O.s.	Left eye
o.m.	Each morning (del latín: *omni mane*)
o.n.	Each night (del latín: *omni nocte*)
OU	In each eye
p.	Parts
p.a.	Active (s) principle (s)
p.c.	After the meals (del latín: post cibos)
P.O.	Oficinal preparation
p.r.n.	In a necessary case (del latín: *pro re nace*)

Part. Aeq.	Equals parts (del latín: *partes aecuales*)
q.	Each
q.4h.	Each 4 hours (del latín: *quartaquaque hora*)
q.d. o q.i.d.	Fourth time daily (del latín: *quarter in die*)
q.h.	Each hour (del latín: *quaque hora*)
q.l.	As much as is necessary (del latín: *quantum libet*)
q.s.	In enough quantity e (del latín: *quantum suficiant*)
Qam	Each morning (del latín: *omni mane*)
Quotid	Daily (del latín: *quotidie*)
QV o QQV	As much as you see
R.	To drink (del latín: *recipe*)
s.o.s.	If is necessary (del latín: *si opus sit*)
s.s.	A half (del latín: *semis*)
Sig.	Singh it (del latín: *signetur*)
Sine	Without (del latín:)
Soluc	Solution
Stat.	Immediately (del latín: *statim*)
Sup	Supositories(s)
t.d. o t.i.d.	Three times daily (del latín: *ter in die*)
Tbsp o Coch. Mag.	1 spoon (15 ml)
ut dict.	Como se indique (del latín: *ut dictum*)

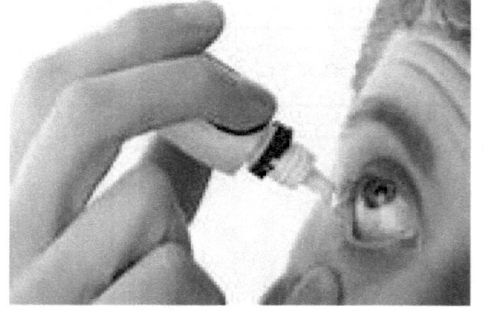

VIAS OF ADMINISTRATION

Abreviaturas	Definición of the VIA
IM	Intramuscular
IV	Intravenous
VB	(the mouth) (rinse, topic)
Vic	Intracavenous
Vinh	Inhalatory
VO	Oral
Vof	Oftálmic
Vot	Otic
VP	Parenteral
VR	Rectal
VSc	Subcutanous
VSl	Sublingual
VT	Topic
VTd	Transdérmic
VV	Vaginal (or Vulvar)

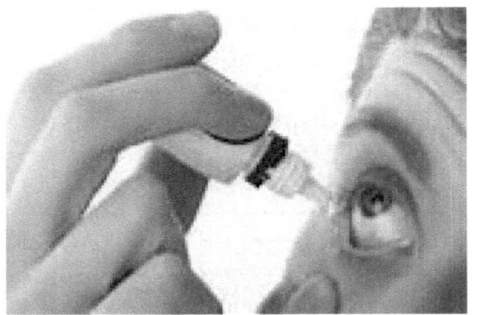

UNITS OF MEASUREMENT

Abreviaturas	Definición
G	Gram
GT	Drop
MCG	Microgram
MCL	Microliter
MEQ	Miliequivalents
MG	Miligram
ML	Mililiter
MU	Internacional Units x 10^6, (millions of UI)
U	Units
UI	Internacional Units
UN	Internacional Unitsx 10^3 (Thousands of UI).

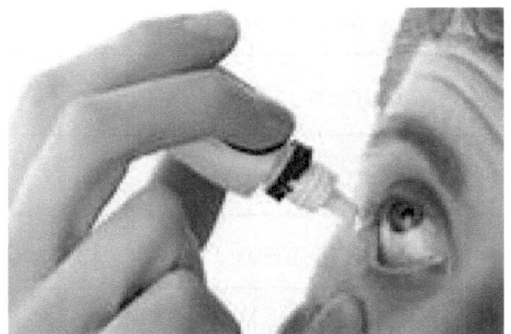

SOME MEDICS ABREVIATIONS AND ITS MEANINGS

Abreviatura Inglés	Significado en inglés
ABCs	airways, breathing and circulation
ACI	acute coronary insufficiency
ACL	anterior cruciate ligament
ACLS	advanced cardiac life support
ACMV	assist-controlled mechanical ventilation
ACO	alert, cooperative, oriented
AD	alternating days
AD	Alzheimer disease
ADI	aceptable daily intake
ADR	adverse drug reaction
AF	atrial fibrillation
AF	amniotic fluid
AH	arterial hypertension
AHD	acute heart disease
AHF	acute heart failure
AID	acute infectious disease

Abreviatura Inglés	Significado en inglés
AIDS	acquired immunodeficency syndrome
ALP	alkaline phosphatase
ALS	advanced life support
AMI	acute myocardial infarction
AP	arterial pressure
ARDS	acute respiratory distress syndrome
ARF	acute renal failure
ASU	ambulatory surgery unit
ATP	attending physician
AV	arteriovenous
AV	artificial / assisted ventilation
BCP	birth control pills
bd.	birth date
BD	blood donor
BD	brain death
BF	blood flow
BI	brain injury
bib.	drink
b.i.d.	twice a day

Abreviatura Inglés	Significado en inglés
b.i.w.	twice a week
BL	blood loss
BMI	body mass index
BP	blood pressure
bpm	beats per minute
BW	birth weight
Bwt	body weight
Bx	biopsy
Ca.	cancer
CBC	complete blood count
CCI	chronic coronary insufficiency
CCU	coronary care unit
CD	cardiac disease
CHD	congenital heart desease
CHF	congestive heart failure
CI	cardiac insufficiency
CI	cerebral infarction
CMD	chief medical director

Abreviatura Inglés		Significado en inglés
	CME	continuing medical education
	CMP	cardiomyopathy
	CMV	cytomegalovirus
	CNS	central nervous system
D	COPD,COLD	chronic obstructive pulmonary / lung disease
	CPR	cardiopulmonary resuscitation
	CRI	chronic renal insufficiency
	CT	chemotherapy
	CT	computed tomography
	CVD	cardiovascular disease
	CVP	central venous pressure
	CVS	cardiovascular system
	CXR	chest x-ray
	DA	degenerative arthritis
	D/A	date of admission
	DBP	diastolic blood pressure
	DM	diastolic murmur
	DNI	do not intubate

Abreviatura Inglés	Significado en inglés
DNR	do not resuscitate
DOB	date of birth
DON	director of nursing
Dx	diagnosis
E	cortisone
EA	enteral alimentation
ECG, EKG	electrocardiogram
Echo.	echocardiography
ED	Emergency Department
EEG	electroencephalogram
EMS	emergency medical service
ER	emergency room
ESR	erythrocyte sedimentation rate
ETT	endotracheal tube
Exam.	examination
FA	fatty acids
FECG	fetal electrocardiogram
FEV	forced expiratory volumen

Abreviatura Inglés	Significado en inglés
FH	family history
FHR	fetal heart rate
FMD	family medical doctor
FUO	fever of unknown origin
Fx	fracture
GA	general anaesthesia
GDM	gestational diabetes mellitus
GE	gastroenteritis
GG	gamma globulin
GH	growth hormone
GI	gastrointestinal
GP	general practitioner
GP	general paralysis
G.U.	genitourinary
HAT	hospital arrival time
HAV, HBV	hepatitis A, B virus
HCT	hematocrit
HD	hemodialysis
HD	Hodgkin's disease

Abreviatura Inglés	Significado en inglés
HF	heart failure
HIV	human immunodeficiency virus
HO	house officer
HR	heart rate
IA	intra-arterial
ICH	intracreaneal hemorrhage
ICN	Intensive Care Nursery
ICU	Intensive Care Unit
ID	infectious disease
IM	internal medicine
I.M.	intramuscular
INJ	injury
IT	intensive therapy
IU	intrauterine
IUD	intrauterine device
IUP	intrauterine pregnancy
I.V.	intravenous
IVF	in vitro fertilization

Abreviatura Inglés	Significado en inglés
LA	long-acting
LA	local anaesthesia
LBW	low birth weight
LD	lethal dose
MAP	mean arterial pressure
MAS	meconium aspiration syndrome
MD	muscular dystrophy
MH	medical history
MH	mental health
MI	mental illness
MI	myocardial infarction
MICU	mobile intensive care unit
NA	not available
NA, N/A	not applicable
NAA	no apparent abnormalities
NB	newborn
NBI	no bone injury
NBP	non-invasive blood pressure
NFR	not for resuscitation

Abreviatura Inglés	Significado en inglés
NG(T)	nasogastric (tube)
NHS	National Health Service
NICU	Neonatal Intensive Care Unit
NIF	negative inspiratory force
NLG	natural latex gloves
nlt.	not lower than
NM	neuromuscular
NM	not measured
NN	neonatal
NOAEL	no observable adverse effect level
NSG	nursing
NSR	normal sinus rhythm
NSS	normal size and shape
NV	neurovascular
OCD	obsessive-compulsive disorder
OOB	out of bed
OR	operating room
OS	oxygen saturation

Abreviatura Inglés	Significado en inglés
OT	ocular tension
OT	occupational therapy
OTC	over the counter
OW	overweight
PA	physician's assistant
PA	posteroanterior
PACU	Post Anaesthesia Care Unit
PAD	preliminary anatomic diagnosis
PALS	pediatric advanced life support
PCP	primary care physician
PD	pulmonary disease
PE	physical examination
PE	pulmonary edema
PIH	pregnancy induced hypertension
PIP	peak inspiratory pressure
PMS	pre-menstrual syndrome
pn.	pain
PNC	prenatal care
p.o.	by mouth

Abreviatura Inglés	Significado en inglés
PP	per protocol
pt.	patient
PTA	prior to arrival
PTL	preterm labor
Px	prognosis
q.a.m.	every morning
QC	quality control
q.d.	every day
q.h.	every hour
q.2.h., q.4.h....	every two hours, every four hours...
q.p.m.	every afternoon / evening
q.n.	every night
q.o.d., q.o.h...	every other day, hour...
RATx	radiation therapy
RD	respiratory disease
RR	respiratory rate
RTI	respiratory tract infection

Abreviatura Inglés	Significado en inglés
Rx	prescription
SBP	systolic blood pressure
Sed rate	sedimentation rate
SS, S/S, S&S	signs and symptons
SSD	syndrome of sudden death
st.	stage of disease
SVC	superior vena cava
SVT	supra ventricular tachycardia
Sx	symptoms
tab.	tablet
TB	tuberculosis
T/D *	once daily
TIA	transient ischemic attack
t.i.d.	three times a day
TLC	total lung capacity
TNM	tumor, nodes, metastases
TS	thoracic surgery
Tx	treatment

Abreviatura Inglés	Significado en inglés
UA, U/A	urinalysis
UA	upper airways
UB	urinary bladder
UC	unconscious
UC	urine culture
UD	undetermined
VS	vital signs
w/	with
WBC	white blood cells
w/c	wheelchair
WD	well developed
WER	weekly epidemiological record
WNL	within normal limits
Wt	weight
XR	x-ray
XRT	radiotherapy
y/o	year old

BIBLIOGRAFIA

1. Abad Gimeno FJ, Pons Cabrera J, Micó Mérida M, Casterá Melchor DE, Bellés Medall MD, Sánchez Pedroche A. Categorías de riesgo de los medicamentos utilizados durante el embarazo. Guía rápida de consulta. FAP, Farmacia de Atención Primaria. 2005.
2. Guía de Prescripción Terapéutica (GPT). Información de medicamentos autorizados en España. Adaptación de la 51.ª edición del British National Formulary (BNF).
3. Guía Farmacoterapéutica de Fisterra. Disponible en: http://www.fisterra.com/medicamentos/ Sociedad Española de Medicina Familiar y Comunitaria, sem FYC:
4. Guía Terapéutica en Atención Primaria. Basada en la Evidencia. 3.ª ed. 2007.
5. Empleo de fármacos en embarazo y lactancia - PAHO.org/ pdf. www.paho.org/.../index.php?...farmacos...embarazo...

6. Categorías farmacológicas en el embarazo - Wikipedia, la. .https://es.wikipedia.org/.../Categorías_farmacológicas_en_ el embarazo.
7. FARMACOLOGÍA DEL PACIENTE PEDIÁTRICO - Science Direct. www.sciencedirect.com/science/article/pii/S071686401630091 8.
8. Guía terapéutica para la APS. Editorial José Martí. Ciudad de la Habana. 1994
9. Farmacología clínica Morón y Levy. Editorial Ciencias Médicas. Ciudad de la Habana 2005.
10. Manual Merck de medicina Interna. 10ma edición. Estados unidos de américa. Sección farmacología clínica. Riesgo beneficio. 2009.
11. Prospectos de medicamentos. Farmacias dispensa.
12. Colegio Oficial de Farmacéuticos de Pontevedra Abreviaturas y Siglas https://www.cofpo.org/index.php/abreviaturas.425.htm.

13. Estandarización de abreviaturas, símbolos y expresiones utilizados en Farmacia.
www.madrid.org/bvirtual/BVCM017661.pdf

14. Más de 200 abreviaturas y siglas médicas en inglés, español y **portugués**
https://www.traducirportugues.com.ar

www.ingramcontent.com/pod-product-compliance
Lightning Source LLC
Chambersburg PA
CBHW030451220526
45464CB00006B/2491